Massage Therapy

Trigger Point Therapy
Acupressure Therapy
Learn The Best Techniques For Optimum Pain Relief And Relaxation

By Ace McCloud
Copyright © 2014

Disclaimer

The information provided in this book is designed to provide helpful information on the subjects discussed. This book is not meant to be used, nor should it be used, to diagnose or treat any medical condition. For diagnosis or treatment of any medical problem, consult your own physician. The publisher and author are not responsible for any specific health or allergy needs that may require medical supervision and are not liable for any damages or negative consequences from any treatment, action, application or preparation, to any person reading or following the information in this book. Any references included are provided for informational purposes only. Readers should be aware that any websites or links listed in this book may change.

Table of Contents

Introduction 6

Chapter 1: Massage Therapy Explained 7

Chapter 2: How to Eliminate Headaches, Tension, and Insomnia with a Head Massage 10

Chapter 3: Improve Your Skin and Circulation With a Facial Massage 12

Chapter 4: Fend Off Sore Throats and Stiff Necks By Massaging Your Neck and Throat 14

Chapter 5: Reduce Shoulder Pain and Stiffness With a Shoulder Massage 16

Chapter 6: Improve Arm and Hand Strength With Simple Massage Methods 17

Chapter 7: Relieving Back Pain 19

Chapter 8: Alleviate Chest Pain, Digestion Problems, and More With Massage 21

Chapter 9: Keeping Your Legs Healthy With Massage. 23

Chapter 10: Alleviate Back and Hip Pain with a Buttocks Massage 24

Chapter 11: Reduce Foot and Lower Leg Pain With a Calves Massage 25

Chapter 12: The Best For Last: Foot Massage 27

Chapter 13: Making the Most of Self-Massage 28

Conclusion 30

My Other Books and Audio Books 31

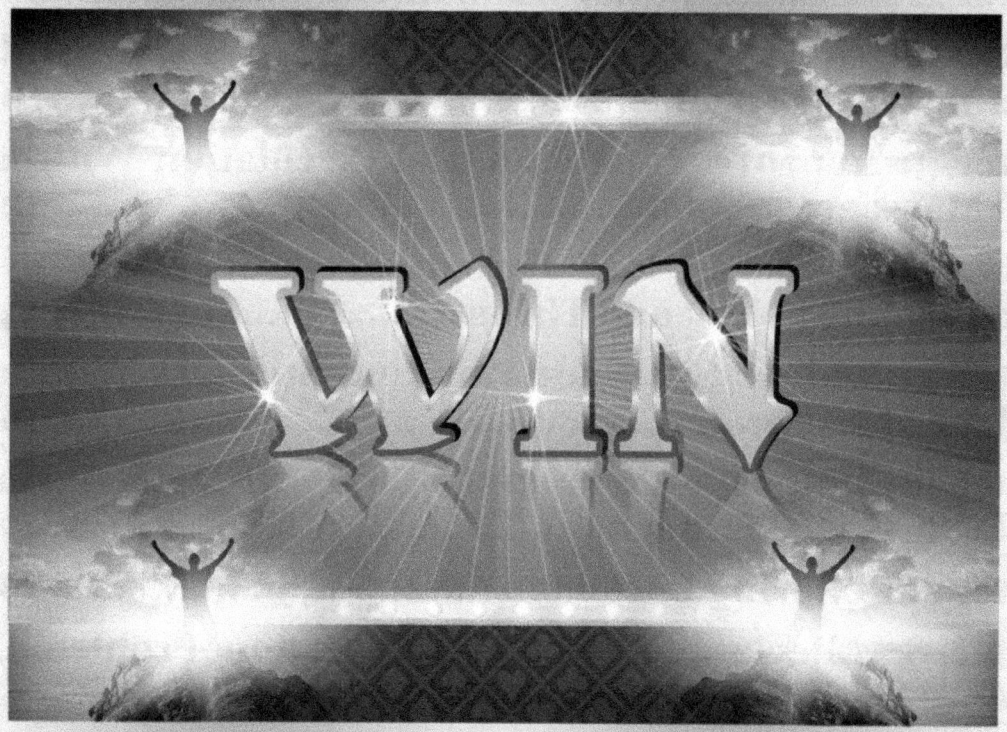

Be sure to check out my website for all my Books and Audio books.

www.AcesEbooks.com

Introduction

I want to thank you and congratulate you for buying the book, "The Best Of Massage Therapy, Trigger Point Therapy, And Acupressure: Learn Exactly How And Where To Massage And Apply Pressure To Yourself And Others For Optimum Pain Relief And Relaxation."

This book contains proven steps and strategies on how to massage yourself and others to eliminate pain, how to locate acupressure and trigger points in your body, and explanations on how massage therapy can work best for you. Furthermore, this book contains many tips, products and suggestions that will help you succeed in mastering massage therapy like a professional. Discover how you can release tension, massage sore muscles, and feel incredible without spending a fortune on professional massages.

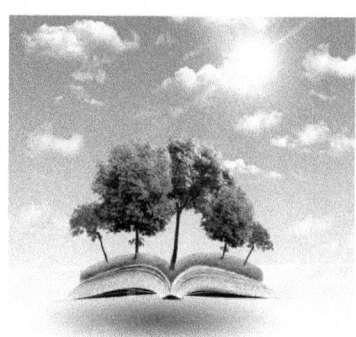

Chapter 1: Massage Therapy Explained

Have your muscles ever ached and felt sore, especially after performing a strenuous activity, working at the computer all day or playing an intense sport? It is natural for our muscles to grow sore after overusing them. You can easily make your muscles and your entire body feel better with the help of massage therapy.

Massage therapy is an excellent way to help your body relax, enhance your physical well-being, and to increase your overall quality of life. Massage therapy has been used for hundreds of years as a treatment method for muscle tension, chronic pain, and a variety of other things.

During massage therapy, another person, usually a masseuse (a licensed massage therapist) asks you what parts of your body need special attention and then applies pressure to those areas with their fingers, hands, elbows, or feet to relieve stress, tension, and pain. The main focus is on your muscles, tissues, skin, and joints. Although people generally pay somebody else to give them a massage, it is possible to learn how to massage yourself and that will be a major focus of this book.

Massage therapy is a very therapeutic process. It soothes muscles, increases well-being, helps with relaxation, releases endorphins and above all, helps with a variety of other ailments, including:

- Anxiety
- Back, leg, neck, body, head, feet, nearly anywhere else, pain
- Carpel tunnel syndrome
- Fractures and dislocations
- Headaches and insomnia
- Muscle tensions or spasms
- Injuries from sports
- Stress conditions
- Post-surgery conditions
- Cancer
- Whiplash
- And more

There are many benefits to massage therapy. First, it is effective in reducing or getting rid of pain in your muscles. Second, it improves the mobility of your joints and your blood circulation. It also helps strengthen your immune system and can even reduce depression. There are almost never any side effects from massage therapy. It is always a good idea to drink a good amount of water after receiving a massage or massaging yourself to flush out any toxins that may have been released by the massage. After many years of trying a variety of different water products, ZeroWater is by far my favorite. You can also save money by buying the filters in larger quantities. ZeroWater filters.

People have been turning to massage therapy for centuries. It dates back as far as the existence of ancient China and is still relevant today. People often enlist in the help of a massage therapist, since it is sometimes hard to massage parts of your body that you cannot reach, such as your back. There are many professional massage places throughout the world, a quick search in your local area will likely pull up a variety of choices. There are also electronic chairs that are programmed to give you a massage. Here is a popular massage chair: Full Body Shiatsu Massage Chair. Be sure to do your research as these chairs do not always fit very small or very large people. Over the long run, a nice massage chair can be very therapeutic and can easily become one of your favorite possessions.

If you are paying somebody else to give you a massage, as incredible as it is, it can quickly get very expensive and may limit you as to how often you can afford to take care of your body. It is always nice to know what you can do on your own to eliminate stress and tension.

The good news, however, is that it is possible for you to give yourself a massage, anywhere on your body and you can save yourself time and money while doing so. This book will cover exactly how to do that by teaching you about the various trigger and acupressure points on our bodies.

One of the first steps in learning about how to treat yourself with massage therapy is to know the difference between trigger points and acupressure points. **Trigger points** are small knots that often form in our muscles. They are called trigger points because they can cause pain in the area of your body that they are in as well as in areas of your body that are connected to that muscle. Often times, trigger points are very painful and sensitive. Trigger point therapy is the process of working these knots out of your body by applying pressure to them. Sometimes, trigger point therapy can be slightly uncomfortable, due to the amount of pressure that can be needed to relieve the pain that these knots can cause. However, trigger point therapy is very effective, especially when combined with acupressure therapy. For powerful knots that can form on the back and lower body, walking on the back, maybe with a support pole, can be very effective for relieving tension in stubborn and tight muscles, especially when done by a professional.

Acupressure therapy is a relatively new healing process that modern therapists have derived from traditional Chinese medicine. Unlike acupuncture, which utilizes needles, acupressure utilizes our hands, fingers, or special devices to work pain out of the muscles. Each one of our body parts have different acupressure points, some of which are connected to others. When combined with trigger point therapy, our bodies can heal quicker and eliminate pain faster.

Why Use Alternative Medicine?

Massage therapy is a type of alternative medicine, meaning that a traditional doctor may not recommend it at first. Some people are simply unaware of the great benefits that alternative medicine can have on our lives. First, massage therapy does not cause any side effects, like a prescribed medication could. Secondly, it is all natural and its benefits legendary. Thirdly, massage therapy is beneficial not only for our physical well-being but for our mental well-being as well, which is another massive benefit. The need for touch by the human race has been well documented by scientists. It has even been shown that babies who have been neglected of human touch ended up getting very sick or dying. In order to be able to perform to your true potential, the human touch can be a greatly beneficial.

Throughout the rest of this book, you will learn how to effectively and easily massage the many parts of your body on your own, or with the help of a partner. You will learn how to identify trigger points and acupressure points for the best results. You will also learn about some great tools that you can use to help you achieve a pain-free body and lifestyle.

Thank you again for downloading this book and I really hope that it will be able to help you change your life for the better!

Chapter 2: How to Eliminate Headaches, Tension, and Insomnia with a Head Massage

Our heads may be hard but they contain plenty of muscles and tissue that you can massage to ease your levels of mental stress. In today's society, it is almost impossible to live without stress. We all experience good stress and bad stress at home, work, and in our personal lives. For many people, it is very difficult to end your night with a peaceful state of mind. Many stress factors can lead to headaches, head tension, mental stress, insomnia, and more. However, by learning how to massage parts of your head and skull, you can eliminate these problems and learn how to get a good night's sleep.

The first step in learning how to eliminate head-related pain is to understand the trigger points in your head. Many headaches, especially tension headaches, start in our trapezius muscles, the large, kite-shaped muscle that covers the left and right side of our neck, shoulders, and upper back. When knots form in this muscle, it is also possible to experience dizziness, jaw pain, and toothaches. The trigger points in our trapezius muscle are located on the sides of the neck, at the base of the hairline, on the tops of our shoulders, and at the tops of our shoulder blades. This YouTube video by expertvillage, How to Find Trigger Points: Trigger Points in the Traps, provides a great visual as to where these trigger points are on our body.

The second step to learning how to eliminate head-related pain is to understand the acupressure points in your head. Our heads contain numerous acupressure points. By knowing where these points are located, you can literally get rid of most headaches, dizziness, and stress. To relieve headaches, insomnia, mental stress, and many other problems you should become familiar with two acupressure points on the head.

The most important set of acupressure points that are located in our heads are known as the GB 20 points. These points help blood circulate into our brains, and if they're blocked, we can feel head pressure, tightness, and even become short-sighted. When these acupressure points are touched, they release pleasurable endorphins into our bodies and can relieve us of stiffness. These two acupressure points are located between the two neck muscles just below the bottom of the ears. To relieve yourself of pain, you should apply pressure to these points with your fingers while taking in deep breaths of air and tilting your head backwards.

Once you are familiar with the trigger points and acupressure points in your head, there are some other basic massage therapy techniques that you can practice to relieve physical head pain and mental stress. One way is to untie your hair if needed, and sit on a chair, preferably in front of a mirror. Keeping your fingers wide open, place your hands on your head. Make sure that your fingers are pointing up. Apply light pressure and move your hands upward. Make sure that your palm and fingers do not release the pressure and stay in contact with your head. Repeat the same process for other parts of the head as well. You can increase or decrease pressure if needed.

Another good method is to place one of your hands on your forehead to stabilize your head as you give a vigorous massage with your other hand. Rub your entire head until you've covered it all. You can then change hands and rub as gently or as forcefully as needed. Another option is to slightly massage your head with your fingers. Move your fingers throughout the head and keep rubbing continuously. Finally, you can gather up strands of your hair in your hands and pull them gently. Keep doing this for different parts of your head, and you should feel a nice tension relieving feeling.

If you do not want to exert your hands and arms to give yourself a head massage, you can use a special device to get the job done. For a head massage, I highly suggest investing in this simple [Head Massager](). It is very inexpensive, small and portable, and easy to use. It doesn't apply much force, but it feels great.

Chapter 3: Improve Your Skin and Circulation With a Facial Massage

Taking care of our face is very important since it is one of our main features. Anybody who has ever received a nice facial treatment knows how important face care can be. Since our face and its muscles are an important part of our body, there are many benefits to getting a facial massage. It has the potential to improve several skin diseases, it improves blood circulation and most importantly, a facial massage is a great way to relax and free your mind of stress. To properly give yourself a facial massage, you must ensure that you know as much as possible about the acupressure and trigger points that are located in your face.

The first step in learning how to give yourself a proper facial massage is to understand the trigger points in the face. The main trigger point located on our face is a muscle called the masseter. This muscle comprises most of our jaw and is what allows us to bite and chew. TrailGuidetotheBody's YouTube video, Masseter, is a great resource for locating your masseter. When there is a knot or complication in this muscle, you could possibly feel headaches, earaches, toothaches, and dizziness. It can also cause a ringing in the ears. Massaging this muscle can help alleviate these symptoms along with possibly helping in problems with people who grind their teeth.

There is a second trigger point in our face called the buccinator, which is located near our masseter, close to the side of the mouth on the cheeks. This trigger point can help relieve gum pain, swallowing pains, and chewing pains.

There is also a third trigger point in our face, located on a muscle called the orbicularis oculi. This muscle is responsible for helping us close our eyes. This YouTube video by Dan Izzo, How the Body Works: Facial Expressions, shows you were this muscle is located. Problems in this muscle can cause eye pain and pain on the sides of our nose. It can also cause difficulties in opening of the eyelids.

The second step in learning how to eliminate face-related problems is to understand our facial acupressure points. By knowing how to locate these points, we can improve our skin health and overall health.

Our first facial acupressure point is called the third eye point. This point is right between our eyebrows, a point on our body in which many people believe our spiritual "third eye" exists. This acupressure point is connected to our pituitary gland, which helps enhance our skin's overall condition. There is a second acupressure point located just below our eye sockets, falling on the cheek bone. Pressing on this pressure point can help in the prevention of acne.

The third facial acupressure point is on either side of the bridge of the nose, at the end of the nostrils. Applying pressure here can help you to relax and fall asleep faster. TheDrSerene's YouTube video [Facial Acupressure Points](#) takes you through a great overview of where these points are on your face, along with a variety of others on your face and head.

There are several ways to massage both your facial trigger points and your facial acupressure points. One way is to massage your masseter muscle gently with your fingers to relive any pain. Another good way to massage your masseter muscles is to put your thumb inside of your mouth while keeping your fingers outside. Press on the muscle between your thumb and fingers. You could also massage your buccinator muscles by putting your thumb inside your mouth with your fingers outside to massage your face gently. To treat the trigger points around your eyes, use your fingertips to massage yourself around the eyes very gently. Finally, you can tap your third eye facial point between the eyebrows for a minute or so to help in getting a peaceful night's sleep. You can also lightly tap this point if you need to gain a few moments of extreme calmness. To get rid of headaches and eye pressure, press on the top of your nose, where it connects to the eyebrows, with two fingers from either side.

One important tip for giving yourself a facial massage is to use a good massage oil that is specifically designed for your face. One of my favorites is [Argan Oil](#). It is an organic product, so it will not make your skin break out. It can help heal acne scars, keep your skin glowing, and is known to help even out your skin tone. Though some people may not enjoy its odor, it is definitely worth using to help keep your skin healthy.

The many ways to massage your face are endless. You can press your eyebrows gently to get rid of any pressure or fatigue or lift your skin up with your palms to "stretch" it out and make it feel good. Another good technique is to place your fingers on the sides of the nose at the bridge and make circular movements. You can also hold your jaws and cheeks with your thumb and fingers while pressing firmly to improve your blood circulation, and to relax your facial muscles.

Chapter 4: Fend Off Sore Throats and Stiff Necks By Massaging Your Neck and Throat

Our necks and throats are two very important and sensitive body parts. It may seem unusual to massage your throat, but it does contain some excellent trigger points that can help eliminate neck pain, throat pain, and help with sore throats, vocal problems, and coughs. Our necks can benefit from a massage because they often become stiff from sitting at a computer too long, from stress, from poor posture, past injuries, or a variety of other reasons. If your neck becomes too stiff and your blood circulation becomes poor, it can cause headaches, anxiety attacks, restlessness, and even dizziness. By learning about the trigger points and acupressure points in your neck, you can help prevent these things from happening to you.

The first step to eliminating neck and throat problems is to understand where these trigger points are. Our most common neck and throat trigger points are located on the lower back part of our heads. There are more neck trigger points located at the tops of your shoulders, on your upper chest, under your chin, behind your jaw, and on either side of your neck. This YouTube video by tensionfreenz, Neck Pain Trigger Pointing, helps you locate your neck trigger points as well as how to locate trapezius trigger points to reduce neck pain.

The second step to alleviating neck and throat problems is to understand the neck and throat acupressure points. There are five acupressure points that can relieve neck and throat pain. The first one is located at the bottom of the skull. The second one is located slightly to the left of the bottom of the skull on the back of the head, the third one is located almost directly below the first one, and right below that is the fourth trigger point. The fifth point is located right in the middle of your neck, right under the base of your head. The most common acupressure point in our throats is located right in the concave spot that is under our Adam's apple. The fifth neck point also serves as an acupressure point that can affect our throats. This short YouTube video, Accupressure: Accupressure Points for Neck Pain by ehowhealth, can help you visualize these points.

There are several ways to utilize these points with massage therapy. First, you can gently yet firmly massage your throat with your fingers to make your voice better and to get rid of throat congestion. You can also slightly massage the point located under your chin with your fingers. Concentrate on the soft muscle that is located in that spot. This is helpful for getting rid of voice problems and it will clear up your voice. You can put your fingers on the either side of your front neck, right in the middle. Push backwards and tap slightly. If you feel a pulse, you are feeling your carotid artery. Just press it gently.

You can also place your fingers on the large concave spot that you will find right under your Adam's apple and apply pressure for 2 minutes. This will help you clear up your throat. It is good for getting rid of a sore throat, a cough, chest congestion, and any heart issues. Another option is to bend your neck and move your fingers to the back of your neck. You will find a jut. This is the pressure point that is helpful with throat issues, neck, and shoulder pains. It can also help in curing a cough. Massage the pressure point with your fingers or hand while moving your fingers in a circle over the pressure point for 3 minutes.

Chapter 5: Reduce Shoulder Pain and Stiffness With a Shoulder Massage

Our shoulders are an important part of our body. They help us lift things, throw things, pull things, and do anything else that requires mobility. Our shoulders can often become stiff and painful when they are injured, dislocated, or torn. Shoulder pain can also occur if you sit in one position for too long. A shoulder massage can improve our blood circulation, which can ease up the pain. Sometimes, shoulder pain is so bad that it requires a deep tissue massage.

The first step to eliminating shoulder pain is to understand the trigger points in the shoulders. Shoulder trigger points are generally found in our shoulder blade muscles, rotator cuff muscles, and prime mover muscles. Our trapezius muscle trigger points can also cause shoulder pain due to their close proximity. This YouTube video, FENIX Trigger Point Therapy Stops Shoulder & Arm Pain by FenixStopsPain, can help you visualize your shoulder trigger points.

The second step in eliminating shoulder pain is to understand the acupressure points in the shoulders. There are around three major acupressure points that are located on our shoulders. You can find these points by drawing an imaginary line from the tips of your ears to the tops of your shoulders. This YouTube video by accupressurepoints, Shoulder & Neck Accupressure Points for Relieving Stress, can help you locate these points.

Since it is often hard for us to reach our shoulders, there are a number of tools that we can use to aid us in finding our shoulder acupressure points. One great tool that I highly recommend is The Original Backnobber. This tool is made from fiberglass and takes the shape of an "S" to help us reach muscles on our bodies that our own arms can't. To relieve shoulder pain, you can simply hook it under your arm. It can also be taken apart, making it a very portable product.

Aside from using specially designed tools, there are some other techniques for easily massaging the trigger and acupressure points on your shoulder. One technique is to use a tennis ball or specially designed massage ball. You can place a ball under your trapezius muscle while laying on it and applying pressure between the ball and the area you want to relieve tension. You can also use your opposite hand to press your shoulder from the top, near your neck. Find the point that gives you the best feeling and then hold for several seconds, and then release. Repeating as necessary.

Chapter 6: Improve Arm and Hand Strength With Simple Massage Methods

Massages to our arms and hands can help us feel happy, relaxed, and can take away any aches and pains that we may develop in those body parts. Hand massages can also provide us with improved finger movements and better wrist movements. Hand and arm massages can also relieve arthritis pains. Best of all, massages to these areas are often quick and easy because these body parts are not as big as other body parts, like our backs and shoulders. We use our arms and hands every day, so it is important to take extra care of them.

The first step to eliminating problems in our arms and hands is to locate the trigger points in them. There are several trigger points for both our hands and forearms. One of the most common trigger points in our forearm is called the flexor carpi radialis muscle. This muscle helps your hands and wrist to flex. The most effective way to massage this trigger point is to apply pressure with your thumb while stretching your wrist. It is good to do at least 10 times or until the pain subsides. This YouTube video, Flexor Carpi Radialis by MessageNerd, effectively shows you how to locate this trigger point.

To the right of the flexor carpi radialis muscle is the flexor capri ulnaris muscle, another trigger point that also helps our hands and wrists flex. You can massage this trigger point by applying pressure with your thumb and holding that pressure for up to eight seconds. You can repeat this action up to 15 times or until the pain subsides. This YouTube video, flexor carpi ulnaris by Jiran Sayadi, will help give you an idea of where to locate this trigger point.

The third trigger point in the forearm is the pronator teres muscle, which can become painful if you overuse a screwdriver or other similar motion. You can massage this trigger point, which is located on your forearm, a little under your elbow, by applying pressure for up to eight seconds while bending your hand. This can be done up to ten times or until the pain subsides. Check out this YouTube video, Active Engagement for Pronator Teres, to locate this trigger point.

Another trigger point in the forearm is the extensor carpi radialis muscle. This muscle helps move your wrists toward your hands. If you are experiencing wrist pain, you should massage this trigger point. You can massage it by placing your fingers an inch away from your elbow, on the inside of your forearm. While flexing your wrist, slowly apply pressure and hold it for up to eight seconds. Do this up to 12 times.

The final trigger point in your forearm is the extensor carpi ulnaris muscle, which also helps move your wrist towards your hand. This point is located about two inches away from your elbow on the inside of your forearm. Apply pressure to this trigger point, holding for ten seconds, and then repeating up to 10 times.

There are also two main trigger points in your hands: the opponens pollicis muscle and the abductor pollicis muscle. Both muscles are connected to your thumbs. To massage both of these muscles, turn your hands so that your palm is facing you. Place your opposite thumb on the fleshy part between your wrist and thumb joint. Apply pressure for up to eight seconds, and then repeat up to five times. Next, bring your thumb to the skin between your index finger and your thumb. Apply pressure for up to eight seconds, repeating this up to five times.

The second step that can help in eliminating problems in your arms and hands is to massage the acupressure points in these body parts. The acupressure points in the arms and hands can help relieve coughs, colds, respiratory problems, and sore throats. Many trigger points are located on the lung meridian, which is located about an inch and a half from the crease in your wrist towards the middle of your hand. See Lung 9's YouTube video [Acupressure massage](#) for a great visual aid. To massage these points, you can massage yourself anywhere on your wrist that you feel pain or discomfort. The best amount of time to apply pressure on these points is up to two minutes.

You can also take a squeezable, rubber ball and hold it tight in your hand. Squeeze the ball and then release it. Continue doing this until you feel tired. This will improve your grip, make your hands strong and it will also increase the blood circulation in your hands and forearms. To relax your forearm, move your finger down from your elbow about 1 inch. Massage this point to relax your forearm. Finally, you can use your thumb to massage the front and backside of your wrist by using an up and down motion. This will improve blood circulation and help keep your muscles active.

Chapter 7: Relieving Back Pain

Back pain can be quite severe and it affects millions of people all around the world. Often times, you can treat back pain with a massage. Back massages are popular and beneficial because they are minimally invasive and do not require any medications to relieve tension and pain. Back massages are also known to help in clearing the mind and as a bonus, massaging the back releases pleasurable endorphins. Back massages are one of the main reasons so many people are willing to pay for a massage. In this chapter, you will learn tips and tricks to help keep your back healthy and pain free.

The first step in eliminating back pain is to understand the trigger points in the back. Our backs are home to several trigger points. The most common one is the erector spinae muscle. The erector spinae muscle is often a primary source of lower back pain and can cause pain in almost every part of the back. This muscle is located on the lower back just above the buttocks. The iliocostais muscle is another trigger point muscle that is connected to the erector spinae muscle. This muscle can also cause stomach pain, leg pain, and neck pain. It is located just below the middle section of the back. Most pain caused by the back muscles is due to poor posture, improper exercise techniques, or overuse. To find problem areas that need attention, run your hand along your back, feeling for areas that are tender or that hurt. Check out this YouTube video by MassageNerd, Erector Spinae Massage Techniques, for a great visual aid. There is also another trigger point located on the gluteus medius which can be massaged to reduce pain and it is located along the lower back just below the hip. See this YouTube video, Gluteus Medius Trigger Points by ModernHealthMonk, to locate this point. Also check out LoseTheBackPain's YouTube video Lower Middle Back Pain – Trigger Point Therapy for more lower to middle back trigger points.

The second step to eliminating back pain is to understand the acupressure points in our back so that you can massage them and apply pressure to them to relieve pain. These points are easy to locate by yourself. The first back acupressure point is located right under your belly button, about an inch below it. Simply apply pressure to this point to help in relieving lower back pain. There are also two more acupressure points on your back, both of which are located two inches from your spinal cord at waist height. They can be fairly hard to locate if you are not familiar with them, but once you find them, applying pressure to them will help in reducing or eliminating lower back pain. For a better idea of how to locate trigger points on your lower back, see this YouTube video by ehowhealth, Acupressure: Acupressure Points for Lower Back Pain. To cure upper back pain, the most vital acupressure point is situated in your sternum area, right in the middle of your chest. The best way to utilize this point is to lie down and apply pressure in this area to help in relieving upper back pain.

One good technique for massaging yourself is to use a ball. Take any ball and press it between your back and a wall. Move your back in circular direction so that the ball changes in direction. You can change the direction of the ball with your hands if needed. You can also use a foam roller to massage your back and get rid of lower back pain. Here is a great foam roller that never loses its shape: Trigger Point Performance Roller. Place the roller on the floor and lie down on it with your lower back on the roller. Ensure that your shoulders, buttocks and all your other body parts are touching the floor except for your lower back which will be lying on the roller. Once the roller is positioned, move the roller up and down your back with the help of your feet. Concentrate on the areas where you feel the most pain.

Another incredible tool that will allow you to apply pressure to your back without the aid of others is the **Backnobber**. This is an incredible product and one of the best things I have ever bought. It does an incredible job of reaching those hard to reach places and relieving back pain and tension.

To give someone else an effective back massage, ask the person to lie on their stomach. Place your hands on the lower back and massage firmly while moving your hands upward, toward their neck. Look for areas of tension or tightness and apply extra pressure to these points. To reduce friction, you can use massage oil. My two favorites are Master Massage and Now Foods Almond Oil. Be sure to massage the spine, lower back, and the shoulder blades.

For more back therapy options, be sure to check out my book: Back Pain Cure.

Chapter 8: Alleviate Chest Pain, Digestion Problems, and More With Massage

In General, our chests and stomachs are not included in a typical massage. However, that doesn't mean that we still do not experience chest and stomach pain. There are trigger points and acupressure points on our bodies that we can massage to help and eliminate discomfort in our chests and stomachs. You can easily practice applying pressure to these points on yourself if you are uncomfortable with other people touching you in these areas.

The first step to eliminating chest and stomach pain is to understand the trigger points that cause those pains. One of the primary trigger points, called the pectoralis major muscle, is located in the top half of your chest. See this YouTube video, pectoralis major by Mari Hopper, for a great visual. This muscle allows us to hug others and bring our arms toward our bodies. On the downside, this trigger point is connected to severe chest pain, similar to that of a heart attack. You can find the pectoralis major muscle by looking for a soft, hollow spot underneath your collarbone. You can apply pressure to this location to relieve pain.

There are also some trigger points located in your stomach area. The most prominent set of stomach muscles that contain trigger points is the abdominal oblique muscle. The first trigger point is located near your ribcage, a few inches below your chest on the left side. This trigger point is connected to both chest and stomach pain. On the left hand side of your body, right beneath your abdomen, are two more trigger points. These two trigger points are connected to pain in the testicles (for men) and pain in the abdomen.

The second step to eliminating chest and stomach pain is to understand the acupressure points in these locations. By locating acupressure points on your chest and stomach, you can relieve yourself from tiredness, respiratory problems, digestion problems, anxiety, and other conditions caused by emotions. Here is a good YouTube video by FirstHealth of Andover PC for acupressure to help with digestion: Indigestion Self-Help with Acupressure.

Two of our chest acupressure points are located on a point called our lung meridian. You can find the first two points by moving your fingers between your clavicle and sternum. These points can relieve problems caused by asthma, chest congestion, and coughs. There is a third chest acupressure point located on a point called the conception vessel meridian. You can find this point by applying pressure to the depression that is between your nipples. This acupressure point can help relieve chest tension, acid reflux, and anxiety.

The next three stomach acupressure points on our bodies are also located along the conception vessel meridian. You can find the first acupressure point by moving your fingers to the middle of your abdomen, halfway between your sternum and your belly button. This acupressure point can relieve digestion issues, heartburn, an upset stomach, and diarrhea. You can find the second acupressure point by moving your fingers to about an inch below your belly button. This acupressure point can relieve bloating and can also fight off tiredness. The third acupressure point that is connected to our stomachs is located two inches above the pubic area, where there is usually a depression. This point is helpful in relieving low energy, diarrhea, and weakness.

There are several ways to massage your chest and stomach area. First, take some massage oil and rub it on your chest and abdomen area. This will help reduce friction. Massage all the trigger and acupressure points that are mentioned above. Another good area to massage is the boundary of your ribs and just underneath of the ribs. This is great for getting rid of stress and for improvement in the digestive system. You can massage your abdomen on both sides. Place your hands on one side of your abdomen and move them up and down pressing gently and then repeat on the other side. For the chest, rub gently throughout the whole chest area with your fingers. This is great for helping to get rid of a cough or reducing chest pain.

Chapter 9: Keeping Your Legs Healthy With Massage

We use our legs every day, so there are many benefits to getting a leg massage. Upper leg massages promote the building of muscles in your thighs, which can help you lose weight. It also helps break down cellulite and can keep your skin looking attractive. There are also many trigger and acupressure points that are located in your upper legs which can help relieve stiffness and pain.

The first step to eliminating upper leg pain and to keeping your legs healthy is to understand the trigger points in this location. Most of the trigger points in our upper legs are located in our quadriceps muscle. This is the large muscle above your knee caps. The most important trigger point in the quadriceps muscle is located a few inches above the knee. By applying pressure to this trigger point, you can relieve pain in your thigh, your knee, and your upper leg.

Another large group of trigger points are located in our hamstring, which is located on the back of the thighs, opposite the quadriceps muscle. The hamstring contains 9 trigger points, but there are 3 primary ones that you can apply pressure to in order to relieve pain. They are called the lower, middle, and the median trigger point. The lower and middle trigger points are located just above the back crease of your knee, and the median trigger point is located just beneath the buttocks. These trigger points can be aggravated by sitting with poor posture or by sitting in bad chair. They can also be aggravated by crossing your legs for long periods of time or from bending too much at the waist. There are some more acupressure points on the inner and middle sections of your thighs. Applying pressure to these points will help eliminate pain, improve blood circulation and can help in keeping your thighs healthy. See this great YouTube video by TrPTherapist for help with locating various trigger points in the legs: Hamstring Pain and Trigger Points.

Here are a few suggestions for massaging your upper legs. Try Lying on the floor face down and place a ball or foam roller in the middle of your upper leg. Then, move your leg up and down by exerting pressure on the muscle. This works great for relieving knee pain and upper leg pain. You can also sit on a chair and place a ball underneath your leg. Move your leg up and down to help get rid of hamstring pain. If you are watching TV or sitting down almost anywhere, you can very easily massage your legs to help relieve pain and tension.

Chapter 10: Alleviate Back and Hip Pain with a Buttocks Massage

A buttocks massage is very beneficial. We use these muscles every day, and when these muscles get tight, they can cause back pain, stiffness in the legs, hip pain, and buttock pain. Also, a buttocks massage can improve your blood circulation and boost your immune system, it can improve the time it takes for your muscles to recover in the event of an injury, and it feels good in general. Some people may be embarrassed by a buttocks massage due to its awkward nature, but if you can get past those embarrassing thoughts, you can help your body improve its functioning. It is never a good idea to totally neglect one or more body parts.

There are 3 main trigger points located in the buttocks on the gluteal muscle. These points can cause pain in your buttock region, your hip joint, and in your lower back. These trigger points are not easy to locate except for the fact that you can trace a point with the help of your finger when you are feeling pain. To locate the gluteal muscle, see this YouTube video about The Gluteus medius Trigger Points and Low Back Pain by TrPTherapist.

Next, you should understand how to locate acupressure points in this area. It is very easy to find acupressure points on your buttocks, since you can easily reach this area of your body. The best way to apply pressure to these points is to press your knuckles into the areas of pain. You can do this while standing up or lying down.

There are some other good techniques for massaging your buttocks. You can lie on your back and place a ball or roller under your buttocks area. Bend your knees and move with the help of your feet. This is a good way to massage your buttocks. You can also massage your buttocks with your hands. Place your hand wide-open on your buttock and rub to help release tension.

Chapter 11: Reduce Foot and Lower Leg Pain With a Calves Massage

Our lower legs—also known as our calves—are very important body parts. They help us move around and they even help us jump. They are very strong muscles that need special attention when they are overused. There are a variety of great benefits from a calf massage. Like most massages, it will improve your blood circulation in this region and reduce scar tissue in the event of an injury. A good massage or trigger point therapy can also help relieve any pain in the area and in the feet.

The first step to understanding how to eliminate lower leg pain is to know where the trigger points are. Since our calf muscles are connected to our ankles, trigger points in our lower legs can also extend to our feet. The first common trigger point location is located in our soleus muscle, which is located at the top of our calves. See this YouTube video, Soleus Trigger Points by Massage Nerd, for a visual aid. The second most common trigger point is located on our posterior tibialis muscle, which you can see in this YouTube video by Richard Finn Tibialis Posterior Trigger Point. Finally, the third most common calf trigger point is located on our gastrocnemius muscle, which makes up the majority of the lower leg. Learn how to locate this trigger point by watching this YouTube video, Gastrocnemius Pain and Trigger Points by TrPTherapist. Rub, massage and apply pressure firmly to all of the trigger points in the area to get rid of pain and discomfort. A good calf massage can help remove heel pain, calf pain, cramps and ankle pain. Also, if you slide your fingers slowly toward the back side of your knee, you will find a soft muscle there. This trigger point can help with depression, stress, low energy, and leg pain.

To find the acupressure points in your calves, simply move your fingers along them until you find the spots that are sore. One common acupressure point is located right under the thickest spot of your calve. There is also an acupressure point along the outer side of your lower leg muscle. The technical names for these two trigger points are "Bladder 57" and "Bladder 58."

There are some other good basic ways to massage your lower legs. One easy way to massage them is to sit on a chair, grip the back side of your leg and apply pressure. You don't have to massage it but you need to squeeze the muscles with a good amount of strength. This will release pressure, pain and stress. You can also lie down on your back and place a ball under your lower leg. Then, move your leg slightly back and forth while applying pressure to get rid of any pain. Rubbing your calf is also very helpful in getting rid of fatigue and leg discomfort. You can massage your calf area with or without massage oil, depending on the situation. The front of the calf needs to be massaged as well. You can massage it gently with your thumbs. Another nice way to massage your front calf is with the help of foam roller. Place the roller on a flat surface and put your front calf on it.

Move your foot in and out so that the calf moves on it. A great foam roller is: Trigger Point Performance Roller.

Chapter 12: The Best For Last: Foot Massage

Our feet are very sensitive body parts, especially since many of us are on them all day long. There is nothing worse than having a pair of sore feet after standing all day. The feet contain a tremendous amount of acupressure points, so a good foot massage is a great way to relieve pain in the feet and other areas of the body. It also helps reduce anxiety, can energize you, can improve blood circulation, and is great for relaxing.

The first step in learning how to eliminate foot pain is to locate the trigger points. Knowing how to find the trigger points in your feet can help you reduce pain in your heels, toes, ankles, and will can help you move better. The most common trigger point in your foot is right in the center, on the arch. You can find this point by placing your hands in between your heel and the ball of your foot. There are also some trigger points near your big toe.

The second step to eliminating foot pain is to understand the acupressure points. A common acupressure can be located in the depression that is found in between the big toe and the second toe. The point where this depression ends is the pressure point. Applying pressure will give you a nice feeling and can remove stress, anger, pain and help with headaches. Another pressure point is located at the bottom of your foot and can be found in between the bones of the second and third toe, about one inch above the base of the toes. Apply pressure here or massage firmly with one finger. This is a great area to relieve pain and calm the mind. There is another pressure point located near the ball of your foot. Applying pressure on this point will have a soothing effect on your entire body. Move your toes back and forth and look for the area that doesn't move on the bottom of your foot. The pressure point is located right next to this area. Check out this YouTube video on [Accupressure: Accupressure for the Foot](#) by ehowhealth for a visual guide.

You can also massage the bottom of your foot and apply pressure on the sole. Massage your heel with both thumbs in small circles. You can either do this forcefully or you can do it gently. Another good area to pay attention to is the very center on the bottom of the foot. Be sure to not forget the toes, and massage every single toe to get rid of pain and stress. Slightly pull the toes and slide your finger between the toes, while moving your toes back and forth with the help of your hand. You can massage your toes all at once with your hand from the bottom as well as from the top.

Chapter 13: Making the Most of Self-Massage

Now that you have learned the ins and outs of massage therapy techniques, the next step is to learn how to enhance your experience.

The first thing you can do is to create a relaxing atmosphere. You can do this by sitting in a dark or dimly lit room. For an added affect you can light some nice candles, burn some incense, or utilize a variety of essential oils. My favorite way to fill a room with pleasant smelling aromas is with an Aromatherapy Essential Oil Diffuser. I never liked the heat based delivery systems of other products, and this one releases a fine mist of sweet smelling aromas and turns off automatically when finished. Some great smelling essential oils you can add to massage oil or a diffuser are: Lavender: known for its relaxing qualities and it smells heavenly too. Eucalyptus is a strong, earthy, but pleasant scented plant that is known to help fight inflammation and reduce swelling. It is thought to clear the mind as well. Marjoram leaves, Peppermint, Chamomile, Cloves, Cinnamon Bark, Sage, Rosemary, Cardamom and one of my personal favorites: Verbena Essential Oil are other fantastic aromatic essential oils that can be soothing as well.

Next, you can play some soothing background music to help you get in a relaxed mental state. You can play anything you want, but I definitely suggest checking out some massage-specific music. My favorite CD is Music For Massage. Another great music CD is: Fairy In The Woods. Nice soothing music can help your mind settle and make the massage session much more enjoyable.

You can also integrate aromatherapy into your massage to help your body relax even more. There is a wide variety of scented massage oils available for you to use on your skin. My favorite kind to use is the Plantlife Aromatherapy Massage Oil. This oil comes in a three pack so you will always have plenty of it on hand. It is made of only natural ingredients and is specially designed for massage therapy. Best of all, these oils smell great, adding to your experience. The lavender scent is my favorite. You can also use massage lotions to help reduce any friction between your hands and your body parts. It will give you a nice feeling as well as soft and smooth skin. My two favorites are Master Massage and Now Foods Almond Oil lotion. It is also always fun to add some of my favorite essential oils to the almond oil or other base oils, for the perfect scent every time.

You can also consider investing in some special massage therapy devices. Sometimes, our own hands are just not enough to work out the knots in our muscles. A great and inexpensive massage therapy tool that I recommend is the Deep Tissue Percussion Massager. Compared to many other deep tissue massage tools, it is cost effective and works great. This tool will give your hands a break and you can use it on almost any part of your body. It comes with four different adjustable heads that you can use to work out specific pains. It is also very light weight and comfortable to hold. Have problems with back pain? Then this is an incredible tool that allows you to eliminate pain and hit pressure points with significant force on your back without the aid of others: Backnobber.

Another one of my favorite massage therapy devices is the Ucomfy Acupressure Foot Massager. As you know from the last chapter, and probably from your own experiences, foot massages are one of the most relaxing and beneficial types of massages due to the incredible amount of trigger points and acupressure points located in the feet. It is a wise decision to go the extra mile in order to make sure that you can provide yourself with an excellent foot massage. This device also uses 24 different infrared heating points for extra healing potential and it has 192 acupressure vibrating points, so you can be sure that your feet will be getting excellent treatment from this device.

Remember in some of the chapters that I suggested using a foam roller to help you out with some hard to reach self-massage techniques? For maximum results, you should consider checking out the Trigger Point Performance Roller. This roller is specially designed for trigger point therapy and is designed to withstand your weight and not lose its shape. It is covered by special bumps and patterns to help you massage any part of your body. It is also portable and relatively inexpensive. I also suggested using a ball for some exercises, too. For those techniques, I recommend using this Massage Ball. Like the foam roller, this ball is also specially designed for trigger point therapy. The ball itself is made to act like a human thumb and is perfect for massaging yourself anywhere on your own. If you would really like to massage or be massaged in comfort, you can invest in a massage table like this one: Professional Portable Massage Table.

While nothing can beat a professional massage, you can save a lot of money over the long term by being able to help yourself in the comfort of your own home on the time frame of your choosing. Be sure to take extra care of your hands and to strengthen them with a grip ball and wrist curls in order to have the power needed in your hands and fingers to truly relieve the pain that can build up in those large muscle group areas. If you can make it a priority to massage yourself on a daily basis, making sure to hit critical trigger points and acupressure points, especially in problem areas, you should be able to live a much happier, healthier, and effective life!

Conclusion

I hope this book was able to help you to learn how to successfully and easily massage yourself and others so that you can save money and feel great at the same time.

The next step is to start practicing some of the techniques outlined in this book. Set aside some time for yourself and check out all the videos, which can help you master the art of massage therapy. Then, start practicing the techniques on yourself. Remember to be consistent—sometimes you will have to work on your problem areas consistently for days at a time in order for them to stay away. Once you begin to see improved results in your body, try these techniques out on your friends and family members. They are sure to be impressed at how great you are at relieving their tension and pain.

Finally, if you discovered at least one thing that has helped you or that you think would be beneficial to someone else, be sure to take a few seconds to easily post a quick positive review. As an author, your positive feedback is desperately needed. Your highly valuable five star reviews are like a river of golden joy flowing through a sunny forest of mighty trees and beautiful flowers! *To do your good deed in making the world a better place by helping others with your valuable insight, just leave a nice review.*

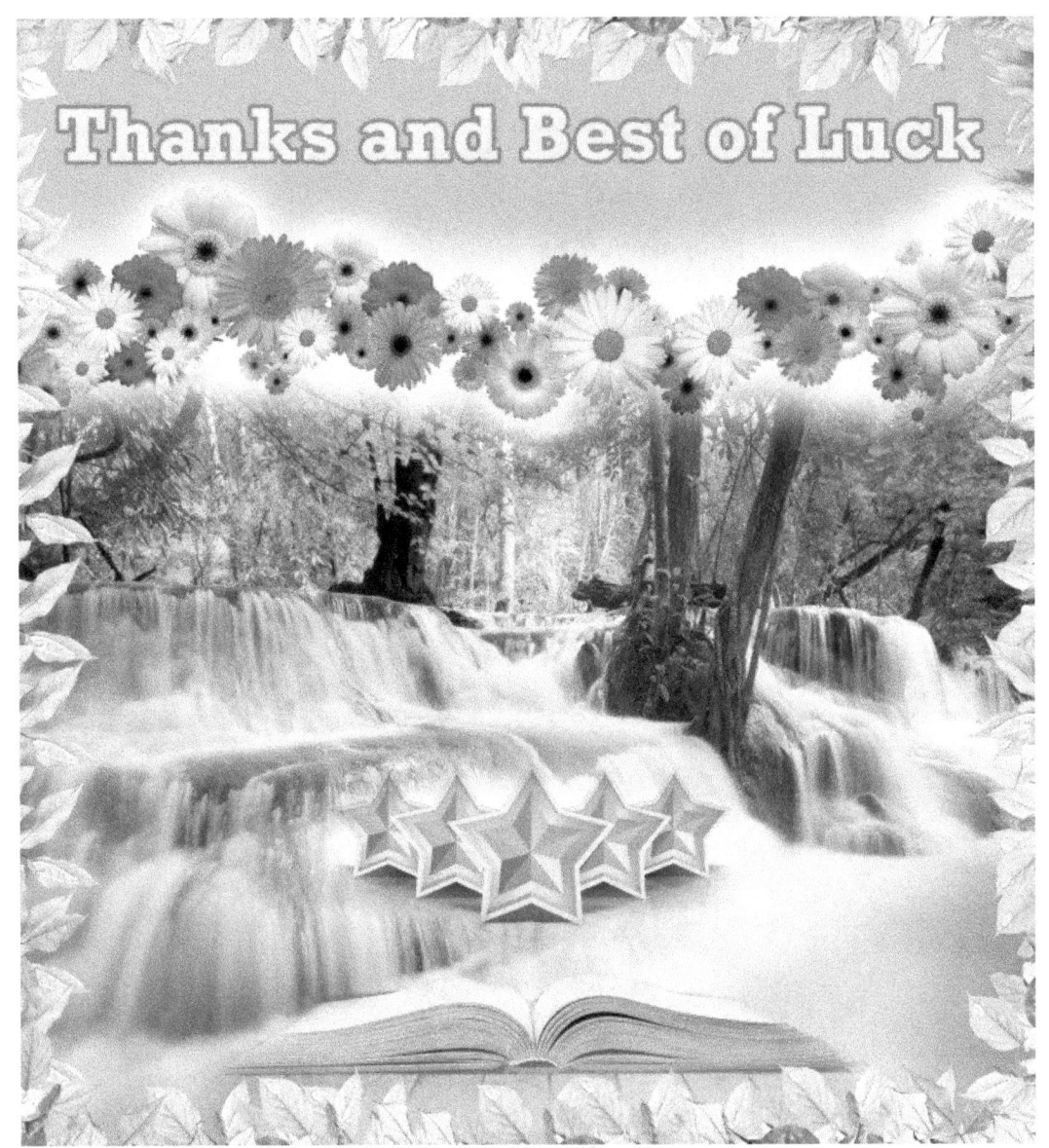

My Other Books and Audio Books
www.AcesEbooks.com

Health Books

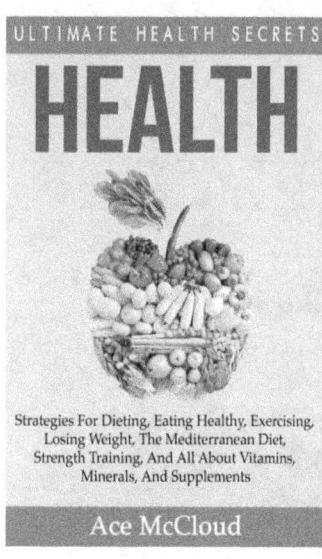
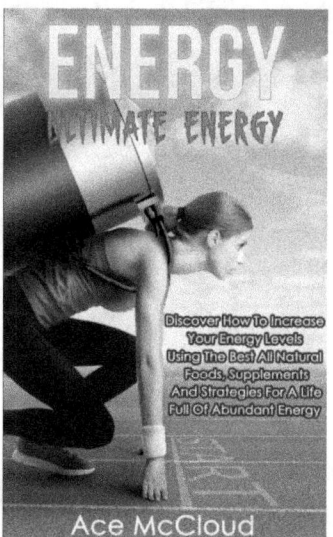
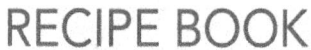
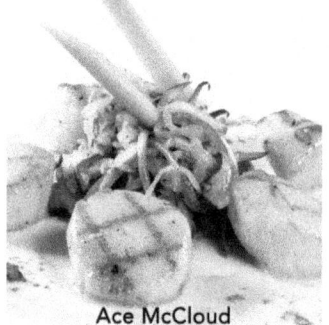
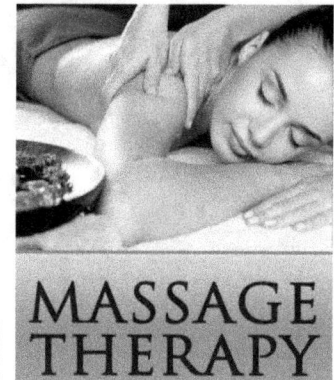
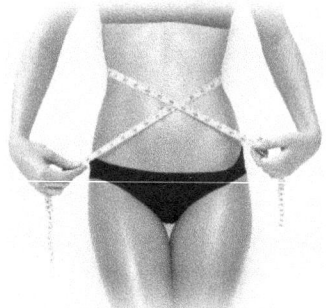
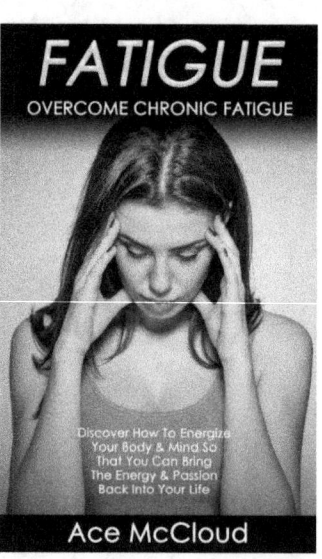

Peak Performance Books

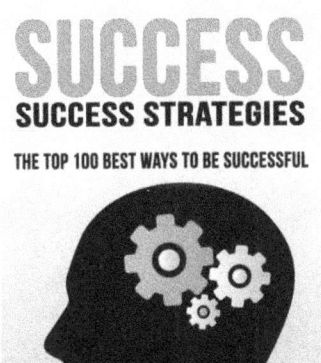
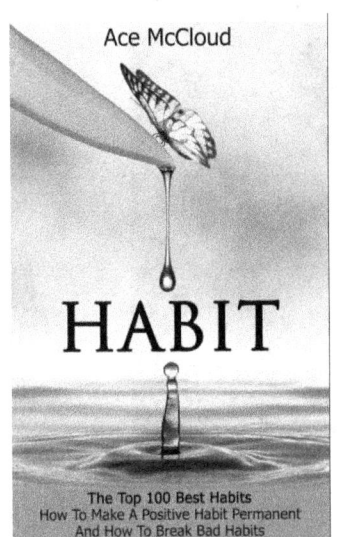
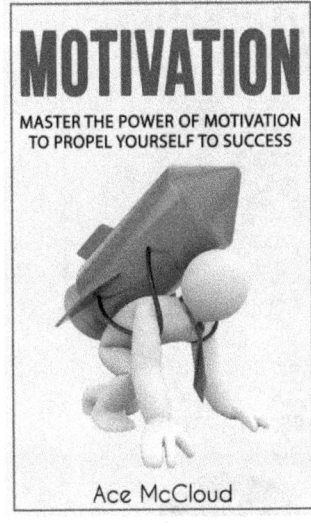
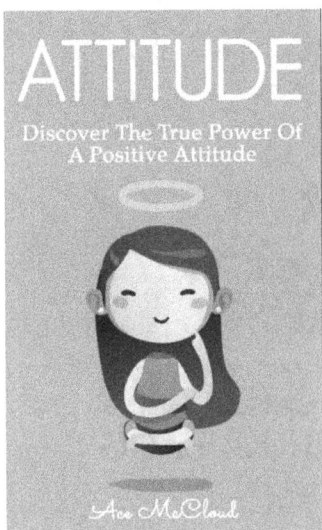

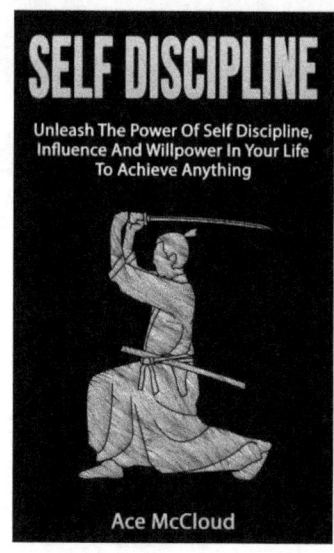 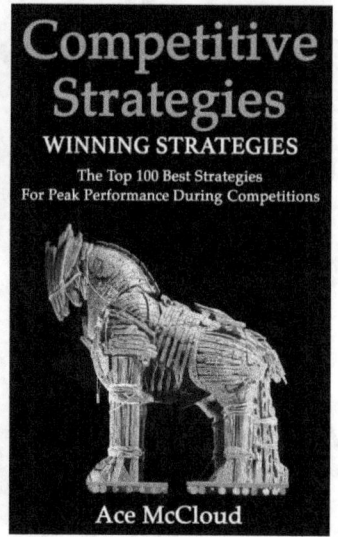

Be sure to check out my audio books as well!

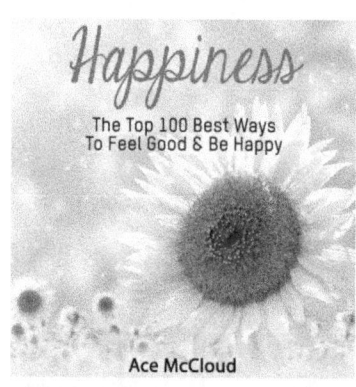 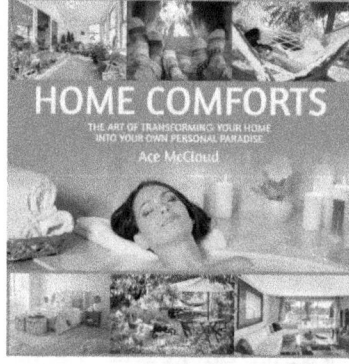 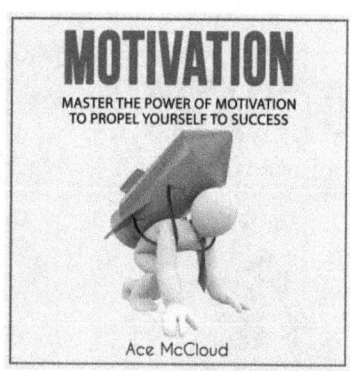

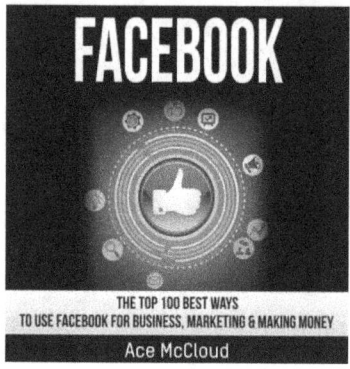 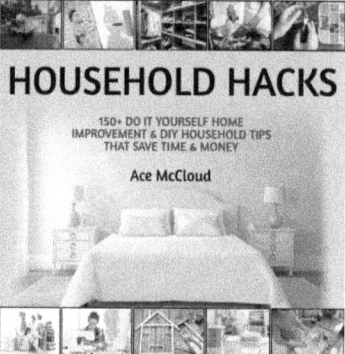 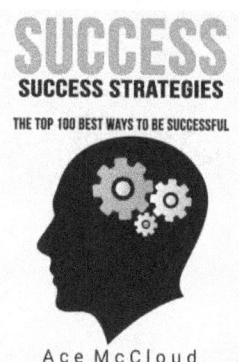

Check out my website at: **www.AcesEbooks.com** for a complete list of all of my books and high quality audio books. I enjoy bringing you the best knowledge in the world and wish you the best in using this information to make your journey through life better and more enjoyable! **Best of luck to you!**